NATURAL REMEDIES
FOR
HIGH BLOOD PRESSURE

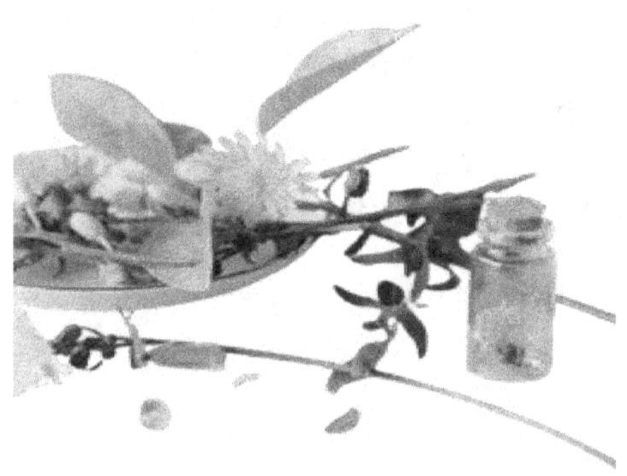

Effective Heart healthy Guide to Naturally Reverse Hypertension, Cardiovascular diseases with Alternative Herbal Medicine, Tinctures, Detox tea and Supplement

DR. BRENDA GRIMM

TABLE OF CONTENTS

INTRODUCTION

Welcome to the enlightening journey within the pages of ***"Natural Remedies for High Blood Pressure."*** As we open this guide to optimal heart health, let me share a story that encapsulates the transformative power hidden within these chapters.

Meet Kate, a friend's aunt on a quest for a healthier heart. Faced with the challenges of high blood pressure, Kate stumbled upon this very book.

Intrigued and hopeful, she delved into the pages, discovering a treasure trove of alternative solutions to address her cardiovascular concerns.

Intrigued by the promises of natural remedies, Kate embraced the various procedures detailed in the book.

She integrated herbal wisdom, explored the world of tinctures, sipped on detox teas, and welcomed the support of supplements into her routine.

The result? A profound positive shift in her heart health.

Impressed by the evident changes in her well-being, Kate became a beacon of inspiration. She couldn't keep this transformative knowledge to herself.

With enthusiasm, she recommended the book to friends and others grappling with high blood pressure.

To her delight, they too embarked on a similar journey and, one by one, testified to the efficacy of the remedies within these pages.

This introduction isn't just a prelude to a book; it's an invitation to witness stories of real change, like Kate's, that unfold within the folds of these chapters.

So, as you embark on this exploration of natural remedies, envision the possibilities for your own heart health journey.

May the wisdom within these pages be the catalyst for positive change, just as it was for Kate and countless others.

Welcome to a realm where nature meets remedy, and where hearts find their path to vitality.

CHAPTER 1

HERBAL REMEDIES FOR HIGH BLOOD PRESSURE

1.1 Overview of Herbal Medicine for High Blood Pressure

High blood pressure, often called hypertension, silently lurks in many lives, posing a serious threat to heart health. As we delve into the world of herbal remedies, we unlock nature's arsenal to combat this silent adversary.

Understanding Hypertension

High blood pressure occurs when the force of blood against the walls of your arteries is consistently too high.

This condition, if left unchecked, can lead to severe health issues such as heart disease, stroke, and kidney problems.

Nature's Pharmacy: Herbal medicine, also known as herbalism, taps into the therapeutic properties of plants to promote health and well-being.

For centuries, various cultures around the world have utilized herbs to address a myriad of health concerns, including hypertension.

Holistic Healing: Herbal remedies offer a holistic approach to managing high blood pressure. Unlike some conventional medications, herbs often work synergistically with the body, addressing not just the symptoms but the underlying causes.

Key Herbal Players

Hawthorn Berry: Known for its cardiovascular benefits, hawthorn berry has been used traditionally to support heart health and regulate blood pressure. It's believed to enhance blood flow and strengthen the heart muscle.

Garlic: More than just a kitchen staple, garlic has been praised for its potential to lower blood pressure. Allicin, a compound found in garlic, is thought to relax blood vessels and improve circulation.

Olive Leaf: Extracted from the leaves of the olive tree, this herb is rich in antioxidants and may contribute to the dilation of arteries, aiding in blood pressure regulation.

Herbal Medicine in Action

Balancing Act: Herbal remedies often work by promoting balance within the body.

Whether through relaxing blood vessels, reducing inflammation, or supporting kidney function, these herbs offer a gentle yet effective approach to hypertension management.

A Word of Caution: While herbal remedies can be powerful allies, it's crucial to consult with a healthcare professional before incorporating them into your routine, especially if you are already taking prescribed medications.

In the upcoming sections, we will explore specific herbs, their properties, and how to integrate them into your daily life to naturally manage high blood pressure.

Join us on this journey into the heart of herbal medicine for a healthier, balanced life.

1.2 Herbs for Blood Pressure Regulation with Ingredients, preparation method and Health benefits

Hawthorn Berry

Ingredients:

Dried hawthorn berries

Boiling water

Preparation:

Place a teaspoon of dried hawthorn berries in a cup.

Pour boiling water over the berries.

Let it steep for 10-15 minutes.

Strain and enjoy.

Health Benefits:

Hawthorn berry is renowned for its cardiovascular benefits. Rich in flavonoids, it's believed to dilate blood vessels, improving blood flow.

Regular consumption may help regulate blood pressure by reducing resistance in the arteries.

Additionally, hawthorn berry is associated with strengthening the heart muscle.

Garlic

Ingredients:

Fresh garlic cloves

Olive oil

Preparation:

Crush and mince fresh garlic cloves.

Heat olive oil in a pan.

Add minced garlic and sauté until golden.

Consume as a flavorful addition to meals.

Health Benefits:

Garlic contains allicin, a compound with potential blood pressure-lowering effects.

Allicin is thought to relax blood vessels, promoting better circulation.

Regular intake of garlic may contribute to reduced blood pressure and overall cardiovascular health.

Olive Leaf

Ingredients:

Dried olive leaves

Hot water

Preparation:

Place a tablespoon of dried olive leaves in a teapot.

Pour hot water over the leaves.

Allow it to steep for 5-7 minutes.

Strain and sip on this herbal infusion.

Health Benefits:

Olive leaf is rich in antioxidants, which may help improve artery function and reduce inflammation.

The compounds in olive leaf are believed to contribute to the dilation of arteries, aiding in blood pressure regulation.

Regular consumption supports overall heart health.

Hibiscus

Ingredients:

Dried hibiscus flowers

Boiling water

Preparation:

Add a tablespoon of dried hibiscus flowers to a teapot.

Pour boiling water over the flowers.

Let it steep for 5-10 minutes.

Strain and enjoy as a refreshing tea.

Health Benefits:

Hibiscus is known for its diuretic properties, which can contribute to lower blood pressure.

It is also rich in anthocyanins and antioxidants, which may play a role in vasodilation.

Regular consumption of hibiscus tea may aid in hypertension management.

Ginger:

Ingredients:

Fresh ginger root

Water

Preparation:

Peel and thinly slice fresh ginger root (about 1 tablespoon).

Boil a cup of water.

Add the ginger slices to the boiling water.

Let it simmer for 5-10 minutes.

Strain and enjoy as ginger tea.

Health Benefits:

Ginger is known for its potential to improve blood circulation and lower blood pressure.

It contains bioactive compounds that may help relax blood vessels, promoting better blood flow. Additionally, ginger has anti-inflammatory properties that can benefit overall cardiovascular health.

Turmeric:

Ingredients:

Ground turmeric or fresh turmeric root

Milk (dairy or plant-based)

Preparation:

Mix a teaspoon of ground turmeric or grate fresh turmeric root into a cup.

Heat a cup of milk until warm.

Add the turmeric to the warm milk.

Stir well and drink as turmeric milk.

Health Benefits:

Turmeric contains curcumin, a powerful compound with anti-inflammatory and potential blood pressure-lowering effects.

Regular consumption of turmeric may contribute to overall heart health and help manage hypertension.

Lemon Balm:

Ingredients:

Fresh or dried lemon balm leaves

Boiling water

Preparation:

Place a tablespoon of fresh or dried lemon balm leaves in a cup.

Pour boiling water over the leaves.

Let it steep for 5-7 minutes.

Strain and enjoy as lemon balm tea.

Health Benefits:

Lemon balm is celebrated for its calming properties, which may help reduce stress and anxiety.

By promoting relaxation, lemon balm tea indirectly supports heart health, contributing to the overall well-being of the cardiovascular system.

Dandelion:

Ingredients:

Dandelion leaves (fresh or dried)

Boiling water

Preparation:

Place a tablespoon of fresh or dried dandelion leaves in a teapot.

Pour boiling water over the leaves.

Allow it to steep for 10-15 minutes.

Strain and enjoy as dandelion leaf tea.

Health Benefits:

Dandelion leaf tea is considered a natural diuretic, aiding in the elimination of excess fluids from the body.

This diuretic effect may contribute to blood pressure regulation.

Additionally, dandelion leaves are rich in potassium, a mineral important for heart health.

Note:

Always consult with a healthcare professional before incorporating new herbs into your routine, especially if you are on prescribed medications.

Incorporating these herbs into your daily life, alongside a healthy lifestyle, may contribute to the natural management of high blood pressure. Remember, consistency is key in reaping the benefits of herbal remedies.

CHAPTER 2

TINCTURES FOR HYPERTENSION

In the world of natural remedies, tinctures emerge as potent elixirs, offering a concentrated form of herbal goodness.

In this chapter, we embark on a journey into the realm of tinctures, exploring how these liquid extracts can become your allies in the quest for managing hypertension.

Unveiling the Magic of Tinctures

What Are Tinctures?

Tinctures are herbal extracts made by soaking herbs in alcohol or another solvent.

This process draws out the active compounds, creating a concentrated liquid that retains the therapeutic properties of the herbs.

They stand as a bridge between traditional herbal wisdom and modern convenience, providing a powerful and easy-to-use form of herbal medicine.

Concentration Power: Tinctures are highly concentrated, packing a punch of herbal goodness in just a few drops.

This concentration ensures that you get the maximum benefits of the herbs without having to consume large quantities.

Long Shelf Life: Unlike some herbal preparations, tinctures have a longer shelf life.

The alcohol acts as a natural preservative, allowing you to keep these herbal allies on hand for an extended period.

Easy Administration: A few drops under the tongue or diluted in water, and you've taken your dose.

Tinctures offer a convenient and straightforward way to incorporate herbal remedies into your daily routine.

2.1 Tinctures for Blood Pressure Management with Ingredients, preparation method and Health benefits

In this chapter, we unravel the potential of tinctures as allies in the pursuit of blood pressure harmony.

Let's explore three herbal tinctures—***Dandelion, Motherwort, and Arjuna Bark***—each with its unique blend of nature's goodness to support the management of high blood pressure.

Dandelion Tincture

Ingredients:

Fresh or dried dandelion leaves and roots

High-proof alcohol (vodka or brandy)

Preparation:

Chop the dandelion leaves and roots finely.

Place the chopped herbs in a glass jar.

Cover the herbs completely with alcohol.

Seal the jar tightly and store it in a dark place for 4-6 weeks.

Strain the liquid, and your dandelion tincture is ready for use.

Health Benefits:

Dandelion is a natural diuretic, promoting the elimination of excess fluid from the body. This diuretic effect may contribute to blood pressure regulation by reducing fluid volume and easing the workload on the heart.

Motherwort Tincture

Ingredients:

Fresh or dried motherwort leaves and flowers

High-proof alcohol

Preparation:

Chop the motherwort leaves and flowers finely.

Place the chopped herbs in a glass jar.

Cover the herbs completely with alcohol.

Seal the jar tightly and let it infuse in a dark place for 4-6 weeks.

Strain the liquid, and your motherwort tincture is ready for use.

Health Benefits:

Motherwort is renowned for its calming properties. By promoting relaxation, motherwort may help reduce stress and anxiety, contributing to a lower blood pressure.

It is also believed to support overall cardiovascular health.

Arjuna Bark Tincture

Ingredients:

Dried Arjuna bark

High-proof alcohol

Preparation:

Crush the dried Arjuna bark into small pieces.

Place the crushed bark in a glass jar.

Cover the bark completely with alcohol.

Seal the jar tightly and let it steep in a dark place for 4-6 weeks.

Strain the liquid, and your Arjuna Bark tincture is ready for use.

Health Benefits:

Arjuna Bark is traditionally used to support heart health.

It is believed to strengthen the heart muscles, improve circulation, and contribute to the dilation of blood vessels, potentially aiding in the management of high blood pressure.

Note: Before incorporating these tinctures into your routine, especially if you are on prescribed medications or have pre-existing health conditions, consult with a healthcare professional.

The power of these herbal tinctures lies in their potential to complement a holistic approach to blood pressure management, including a healthy lifestyle and regular medical check-ups.

Embrace the synergy of nature and science on your journey to optimal heart health.

CHAPTER 3

DETOX TEA FOR

CARDIOVASCULAR HEALTH

3.1 Detoxification and Heart Health

In the hustle and bustle of modern life, our bodies often bear the brunt of daily stresses and environmental toxins.

Enter the world of detox teas—a soothing elixir that not only comforts the soul but also provides a natural boost to your cardiovascular health.

Understanding Detoxification

Before we dive into the realm of detox teas, let's unravel the concept of detoxification. Our bodies have remarkable self-cleaning mechanisms, primarily carried out by the liver and kidneys.

These organs work tirelessly to filter out impurities and ensure the smooth functioning of our internal systems.

The Detox Dilemma: In our fast-paced world, the body's natural detox processes can sometimes use a helping hand. Environmental pollutants, processed foods, and stress can overload our detoxification systems. This is where the magic of detox teas comes into play.

Detox Teas: Nature's Cleansing Brew

Ingredients Matter: Detox teas are crafted from a symphony of herbs, each chosen for its unique properties. These may include dandelion, nettle, burdock, and other cleansing herbs. Blended together, they create a potent infusion designed to support the body's natural detox pathways.

Gentle Cleansing: Unlike aggressive detox trends, detox teas offer a gentle nudge to the body's cleansing mechanisms. They hydrate, soothe, and infuse your system with botanical goodness, making the detoxification process a delightful and nourishing experience.

The Heart-Health Connection

How does detox tea relate to heart health? The connection lies in the intricate dance between detoxification and cardiovascular well-being.

Reducing Inflammation: Many herbs found in detox teas boast anti-inflammatory properties.

By reducing inflammation, these teas may indirectly contribute to heart health.

Chronic inflammation is a risk factor for cardiovascular diseases, and keeping it in check is a key component of a heart-healthy lifestyle.

Supporting Blood Flow: Certain herbs in detox teas, like hibiscus and ginger, are known for their potential to support healthy blood circulation.

This, in turn, assists the heart in its vital pumping role, maintaining optimal blood pressure levels.

Antioxidant Boost: Detox teas are often rich in antioxidants, which combat oxidative stress. Oxidative stress is linked to cardiovascular issues, and the antioxidants in these teas act as warriors, defending your heart from potential harm.

Choosing Your Detox Tea Wisely

As you embark on your journey to cardiovascular health with detox teas, it's essential to choose blends wisely.

Opt for teas that align with your personal preferences and health goals. Whether you enjoy the soothing embrace of chamomile or the invigorating kick of peppermint, there's a detox tea out there for you.

In the upcoming sections, we'll explore specific herbs and blends, unveiling the secrets of crafting your own heart-loving detox teas.

Let the journey to a revitalized cardiovascular system begin, one comforting sip at a time.

3.2 Homemade Detox Tea Recipes with Ingredients, preparation method and Health benefits

Get ready to embark on a journey of flavor and well-being with these homemade detox tea recipes.

Crafted with care and infused with heart-loving ingredients, these blends are not only delicious but also tailored to support your cardiovascular health.

Green Tea and Lemon Detox

Ingredients:

1 green tea bag or 1 teaspoon of loose green tea leaves

1 slice of fresh lemon

1 teaspoon of honey (optional)

1 cup of hot water

Preparation:

Steep the green tea in hot water for 3-5 minutes.

Squeeze the juice from the lemon slice into the tea.

Add honey if desired and stir well.

Health Benefits:

Heart-Boosting Antioxidants: Green tea is rich in catechins, powerful antioxidants that may contribute to heart health by reducing inflammation and supporting healthy blood vessels.

Refreshing Citrus Kick: Lemon adds a burst of vitamin C, promoting overall cardiovascular well-being.

Cinnamon and Ginger Infusion

Ingredients:

1 cinnamon stick or 1 teaspoon of ground cinnamon

1 teaspoon of freshly grated ginger

1 teaspoon of honey (optional)

1 cup of hot water

Preparation:

Place the cinnamon stick and grated ginger in a cup.

Pour hot water over the ingredients.

Let it steep for 5-7 minutes.

Remove the cinnamon stick or strain the tea.

Add honey if desired and enjoy.

Health Benefits:

Anti-Inflammatory Power: Cinnamon and ginger are known for their anti-inflammatory properties, potentially reducing inflammation that contributes to cardiovascular issues.

Warmth and Comfort: This infusion provides a comforting warmth that can soothe and relax, contributing to overall heart health.

Hibiscus and Mint Blend

Ingredients:

1 hibiscus tea bag or 1 tablespoon of dried hibiscus petals

Fresh mint leaves

1 teaspoon of honey (optional)

1 cup of hot water

Preparation:

Steep the hibiscus tea bag or petals in hot water for 5-7 minutes.

Add fresh mint leaves to the tea.

Let it steep for an additional 2-3 minutes.

Remove the tea bag or strain the tea.

Add honey if desired and savor the blend.

Health Benefits:

Lowering Blood Pressure: Hibiscus is recognized for its potential to lower blood pressure by relaxing blood vessels.

Cooling Minty Freshness: Mint adds a refreshing element, making this blend a delightful and heart-healthy treat.

Note: Feel free to adjust the ingredients and quantities based on your taste preferences.

These homemade detox teas offer not only a delightful sensory experience but also a sip toward a healthier cardiovascular system.

Enjoy the journey to heart wellness, one homemade blend at a time.

CHAPTER 4

SUPPLEMENTS TO SUPPORT HEART FUNCTION

The Role of Supplements in Cardiovascular Health

In the intricate dance of well-being, our hearts take center stage, orchestrating the rhythm of life.

As we delve into the realm of supplements, we unlock a treasure trove of nutrients that can be instrumental in supporting and fortifying our cardiovascular health.

Understanding the Harmony of Cardiovascular Health

Before we explore the specific supplements, let's unravel the complex composition of cardiovascular health.

The heart, arteries, veins, and the circulatory system form a dynamic network, ensuring the steady flow of oxygen and nutrients to every cell in our bodies.

This harmony requires a balanced blend of various factors, including diet, exercise, and the right nutrients.

While a healthy diet and lifestyle form the foundation of cardiovascular well-being, supplements can act as supportive elements, enhancing the overall balance.

They offer a convenient and targeted way to ensure that our bodies receive essential nutrients that might be challenging to obtain through diet alone.

Key Nutrients in Cardiovascular Health Supplements

1. Omega-3 Fatty Acids:

Source: Found in fish oil, flaxseed oil, and chia seeds.

Role: Omega-3s are known for their heart-protective properties, potentially reducing inflammation, lowering blood pressure, and supporting overall heart health.

2. Coenzyme Q10 (CoQ10):

Source: Available in small amounts in certain foods, also found in supplement form.

Role: CoQ10 is a vital antioxidant that supports energy production in cells, potentially aiding in maintaining a healthy heart.

3. Magnesium:

Source: Abundant in green leafy vegetables, nuts, and seeds.

Role: Magnesium plays a crucial role in maintaining normal heart rhythm, supporting muscle function, and regulating blood pressure.

4. Vitamin D:

Source: Obtained from sunlight, fatty fish, and fortified foods.

Role: Vitamin D is linked to heart health, potentially helping to regulate blood pressure and reduce inflammation.

The Synergy of a Holistic Approach

Supplements, when integrated into a holistic approach to health, can contribute to the overall well-being of your cardiovascular system.

However, it's important to note that supplements are not a one-size-fits-all solution.

Individual needs may vary, and consulting with a healthcare professional is crucial to tailor a supplement regimen to your specific health requirements.

In the chapters that follow, we will explore each supplement in detail, understanding its unique contribution to cardiovascular health.

Together, let's embark on a journey to fortify the heart's balance, ensuring that each beat resonates with vitality and resilience.

Essential Nutrients for Hypertension and Optimal Cardiovascular Health

As we navigate the landscape of heart health, understanding the pivotal role of essential nutrients becomes paramount, especially for those grappling with high blood pressure.

In this chapter, we unravel the power of specific supplements and how their proper incorporation can pave the way for a healthier cardiovascular journey.

1. Omega-3 Fatty Acids:

Source: Found in fatty fish, flaxseeds, and walnuts.

Role: Omega-3s exhibit anti-inflammatory properties, potentially aiding in reducing blood pressure and supporting heart health.

2. Coenzyme Q10 (CoQ10):

Source: Present in small amounts in organ meats and seafood, available as a supplement.

Role: CoQ10 acts as a potent antioxidant, supporting energy production in cells and contributing to overall heart function.

3. Magnesium:

Source: Abundant in leafy greens, nuts, and whole grains.

Role: Magnesium plays a crucial role in regulating blood pressure, supporting muscle function, and contributing to the overall health of the cardiovascular system.

4. Vitamin D:

Source: Obtained from sunlight, fatty fish, and fortified foods.

Role: Vitamin D is associated with blood pressure regulation and reducing inflammation, contributing to a healthier heart.

1. Dietary Changes:

Integrate omega-3-rich foods like salmon, chia seeds, and flaxseeds into your diet.

Include magnesium-rich foods such as spinach, almonds, and whole grains.

Consume vitamin D sources like fatty fish, fortified dairy, and egg yolks.

2. Supplementation:

Consult with a healthcare professional to determine appropriate supplement dosages.

Choose high-quality supplements for Omega-3s, CoQ10, magnesium, and vitamin D, ensuring they complement your diet.

3. Lifestyle Adjustments:

Engage in regular physical activity to support heart health.

Manage stress through practices like meditation and deep breathing, contributing to blood pressure regulation.

4. Regular Monitoring:

Work closely with healthcare providers to monitor blood pressure levels.

Adjust nutrient intake based on individual needs and health goals.

A Personalized Approach to Cardiovascular Wellness

Remember, the journey to optimal cardiovascular health is unique for each individual. What works for one may differ for another.

Embrace a personalized approach by consulting with healthcare professionals, incorporating essential nutrients into your lifestyle, and consistently monitoring your progress.

Together, let's embark on a path towards better cardiovascular health, armed with the knowledge of essential nutrients and a commitment to well-being.

Through mindful choices and
embracing natural solutions,
you have the strength to reverse
the tide of high blood pressure
and reclaim your health

CHAPTER 5

RECIPES FOR HEART HEALTH

Delicious and Nutrient-Packed Meals

In this chapter, we embark on a culinary journey designed to nourish your heart and delight your taste buds.

These recipes are more than just meals; they are a celebration of flavor and well-being.

Each dish is carefully crafted to include heart-loving ingredients, prepared with love, and infused with health benefits.

5.1 Grilled Salmon with Quinoa and Roasted Vegetables

Ingredients:

Salmon fillets

Quinoa

Assorted vegetables (bell peppers, zucchini, cherry tomatoes)

Olive oil

Lemon

Garlic

Fresh herbs (such as thyme or rosemary)

Salt and pepper

Preparation:

Marinate salmon with olive oil, lemon juice, minced garlic, fresh herbs, salt, and pepper.

Cook quinoa according to package instructions.

Toss vegetables in olive oil, salt, and pepper, then roast until tender.

Grill salmon until cooked through.

Serve grilled salmon over a bed of quinoa, accompanied by roasted vegetables.

Health Benefits:

Omega-3 Fatty Acids: Salmon is rich in omega-3s, supporting heart health and reducing inflammation.

Quinoa: A nutrient-dense grain with protein, fiber, and various vitamins and minerals.

Vegetables: Packed with antioxidants, fiber, and essential nutrients, promoting overall cardiovascular well-being.

5.2 Spinach and Berry Salad with Grilled Chicken

Ingredients:

Chicken breast

Fresh spinach leaves

Mixed berries (strawberries, blueberries, raspberries)

Feta cheese

Walnuts

Balsamic vinaigrette

Olive oil

Salt and pepper

Preparation:

Grill chicken breast until fully cooked.

Combine fresh spinach, mixed berries, crumbled feta, and chopped walnuts in a bowl.

Slice grilled chicken and add to the salad.

Drizzle with balsamic vinaigrette and olive oil.

Season with salt and pepper to taste.

Health Benefits:

Lean Protein: Grilled chicken provides lean protein for muscle health.

Berries: Rich in antioxidants that support heart health.

Spinach: High in vitamins, minerals, and fiber, contributing to overall cardiovascular well-being.

5.3 Quinoa-Stuffed Bell Peppers with Black Beans and Avocado

Ingredients:

Bell peppers

Cooked quinoa

Black beans (canned, drained, and rinsed)

Cherry tomatoes

Red onion

Avocado

Cilantro

Lime juice

Cumin

Chili powder

Salt and pepper

Preparation:

Preheat the oven and prepare bell peppers.

In a bowl, mix quinoa, black beans, diced tomatoes, chopped red onion, diced avocado, and chopped cilantro.

Season with lime juice, cumin, chili powder, salt, and pepper.

Stuff the bell peppers with the quinoa mixture.

Bake until peppers are tender.

Health Benefits:

Quinoa: A protein-rich grain providing essential amino acids.

Black Beans: High in fiber, promoting heart health and aiding in blood sugar control.

Avocado: Rich in heart-healthy monounsaturated fats and potassium.

These recipes aren't just meals; they're a gesture of self-care.

As you savor these delicious creations, remember that nurturing your heart can be a flavorful and joyful experience.

Embrace the journey to heart health one delightful bite at a time.

CHAPTER 6

MIND-BODY CONNECTION FOR HIGH BLOOD PRESSURE MANAGEMENT

In the pursuit of holistic well-being, the mind-body connection emerges as a powerful ally in the management of high blood pressure.

This chapter delves into stress management techniques and explores the transformative impact of meditation and relaxation on fostering a healthy heart.

i. Stress Management Techniques

Understanding the Stress-Blood Pressure Link

Stress, the ubiquitous companion of modern life, can exert a significant influence on our blood pressure.

Chronic stress triggers the body's "fight or flight" response, leading to increased heart rate and blood pressure.

Recognizing and managing stress is a pivotal step towards achieving optimal cardiovascular health.

1. Deep Breathing

Inhale deeply through your nose, expanding your diaphragm.

Exhale slowly through pursed lips, allowing tension to melt away.

Repeat for several minutes to promote relaxation and lower stress hormones.

2. Progressive Muscle Relaxation (PMR)

Systematically tense and then relax different muscle groups.

Start from your toes, working your way up to your head.

This technique promotes overall relaxation and reduces muscle tension associated with stress.

3. Mindfulness and Grounding Techniques

Engage in mindful activities, such as focusing on your breath or observing your surroundings without judgment.

Ground yourself in the present moment to alleviate the impact of stressors.

Consistency is Key: Integrate these techniques into your daily routine to build resilience against stress.

Personalize Your Approach: Explore different methods to discover what works best for you.

Create Relaxation Rituals: Establish calming rituals during high-stress periods to proactively manage tension.

ii. Meditation and Relaxation for a Healthy Heart

The Healing Power of Meditation

Meditation goes beyond stress reduction; it's a transformative practice that nurtures the mind-body connection.

By fostering a sense of calm and promoting mindfulness, meditation can contribute significantly to cardiovascular health.

1. Guided Imagery Meditation

Envision a peaceful scene, engaging all your senses.

Breathe deeply and immerse yourself in the calming imagery.

This technique reduces stress and promotes relaxation.

2. Loving-Kindness Meditation

Cultivate feelings of love and compassion.

Extend these feelings first to yourself and then to others.

This practice enhances emotional well-being and reduces stress.

3. Mindful Walking

Take a leisurely walk, focusing on each step and your surroundings.

Engage your senses and bring attention to the present moment.

Walking meditation can be a gentle way to enhance mindfulness.

Embracing Relaxation Techniques for Heart Health

Regular Practice: Dedicate time to meditation and relaxation each day for cumulative benefits.

Mindful Moments: Infuse mindfulness into everyday activities, cultivating a state of calm awareness.

Explore Techniques: Experiment with various meditation styles to find what resonates with you.

As we explore the mind-body connection, we recognize that nurturing our mental and emotional well-being is integral to cardiovascular health.

By incorporating stress management techniques and embracing the practice of meditation and relaxation, we empower ourselves on the journey to a heart that beats with vitality and harmony.

In the garden of well-being,
cultivate your health with the
seeds of natural remedies.

Each choice you make towards a
healthier lifestyle is a step closer
to reversing high blood pressure.

Your journey to wellness is
powered by your own commitment

CHAPTER 7

CREATING A HOLISTIC HEART-HEALTHY PLAN

7.1 Integrating Natural Remedies into Daily Life

As we craft a holistic heart-healthy plan, the integration of natural remedies emerges as a cornerstone in nurturing cardiovascular well-being.

This chapter unveils practical ways to seamlessly weave these remedies into your daily life, fostering a harmonious balance between nature and nurture.

Incorporating Herbal Remedies into Your Routine

1. Herbal Teas

Infuse your day with the goodness of hawthorn berry, garlic, olive leaf, and hibiscus teas.

Replace your regular beverages with these heart-supporting elixirs.

Sip and savor the natural benefits while hydrating your body.

2. Herb-Infused Meals

Experiment with incorporating heart-friendly herbs into your cooking.

Add garlic and olive oil to your dishes for both flavor and health benefits.

Embrace the culinary artistry of herbs like thyme, rosemary, and basil.

3. Tinctures for Convenience

Integrate tinctures such as dandelion, motherwort, and arjuna bark into your daily routine.

Mix them into your morning beverages or take them directly for a quick and convenient dosage.

Cultivating Herbal Wellness as a Lifestyle

Consistency Matters: Make herbal remedies a consistent part of your routine for sustained benefits.

Explore Combinations: Experiment with combining different herbs to tailor your wellness approach.

Mindful Consumption: Be attentive to how your body responds, allowing you to adjust and refine your regimen.

7.2 Monitoring Blood Pressure Progress

i. Importance of Regular Check-ups

Routine check-ups serve as the compass in navigating your heart health journey.

Regular visits to your healthcare provider are essential for assessing your blood pressure, tracking overall health, and making informed decisions about your well-being.

Key Aspects of Regular Check-ups

Blood Pressure Measurement: Regular monitoring provides a snapshot of your cardiovascular health.

Medication Adjustments: Healthcare professionals can modify your treatment plan based on your progress and changing health needs.

Early Detection: Regular check-ups enable the early identification of potential issues, allowing for timely intervention.

ii. Tracking Lifestyle Changes

As you embark on lifestyle modifications, tracking your progress becomes a valuable tool.

This involves monitoring not only your blood pressure but also the shifts in your daily habits that contribute to heart health.

Effective Tracking Strategies

Keep a Journal: Record your daily activities, diet, exercise, and herbal remedy intake.

Use Technology: Leverage apps and devices to monitor blood pressure, track physical activity, and set reminders for medications.

Celebrate Milestones: Acknowledge and celebrate positive changes, fostering motivation for continued progress.

Informed Decision-Making: Regular check-ups
provide data for informed health decisions.

Motivation and Accountability: Tracking
progress cultivates a sense of accomplishment and
accountability.

Holistic Health Awareness: Monitoring extends
beyond numbers, encompassing lifestyle shifts and
holistic well-being.

In creating a holistic heart-healthy plan, the
integration of natural remedies and vigilant
monitoring form the pillars of a robust foundation.

Embrace this journey as a personal commitment to
vitality and well-being, where each herbal infusion and
every lifestyle adjustment contributes to the symphony
of a heart that beats with resilience and joy.

Every healthy choice you make, every step towards nature's remedies, is a step towards transforming your high blood pressure.

Believe in the resilience of your own well-being

CONCLUSION

As we wrap up this helpful guide, ***"Natural Remedies for High Blood Pressure,"*** let's take a moment to think about what we've learned.

We've explored different ways to keep our hearts healthy by using natural remedies like herbs, tinctures, detox teas, and supplements.

Think of herbs like hawthorn berry, garlic, and olive leaf as heart superheroes. Tinctures, such as dandelion, motherwort, and arjuna bark, are like powerful potions that support our heart health.

Detox teas and supplements act like friendly allies, helping us in our quest for a healthier heart.

But it's not just about the physical stuff—like herbs and teas. We've also talked about how our thoughts and feelings are connected to our heart health.

Techniques to manage stress, the calmness of meditation, and the way our mind and body work together are all part of our plan for a healthy heart.

As you finish reading, remember that this journey to a healthy heart doesn't have to be complicated.

Regular check-ups and keeping track of the changes you make in your life are like having a guide on your journey. They help you make smart choices and understand how your heart is doing.

So, as you go on with your day, think of each small choice you make as a way to paint a picture of a healthy and happy heart.

This guide is here to inspire you, like a map leading you to a heart that's strong and full of life. It's not just about fixing high blood pressure; it's about living a good life with a happy and healthy heart.

Cheers to your heart's adventure and all the exciting chapters ahead!

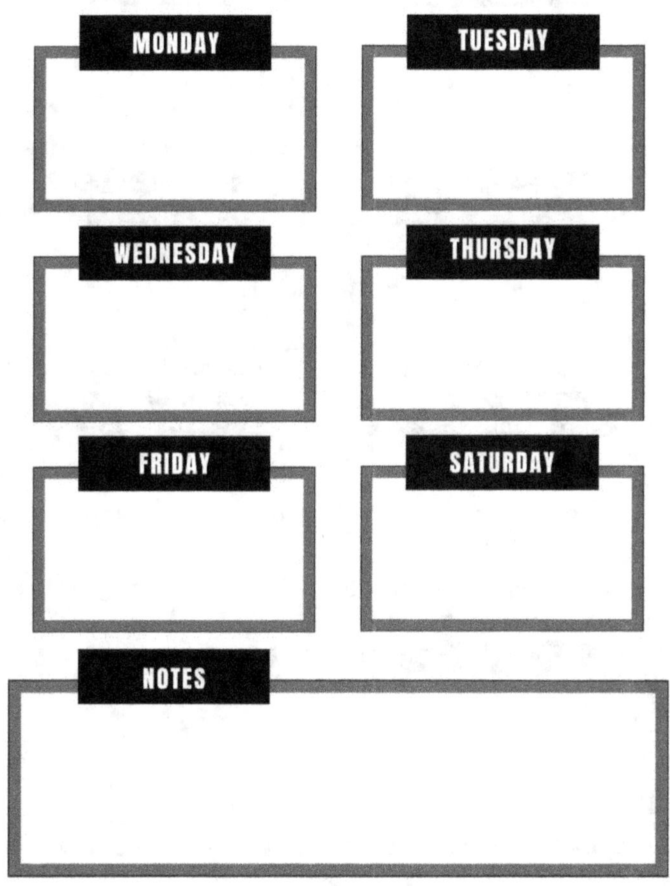
HERBAL RECIPE PLANNER
DATE :
MONDAY
TUESDAY
WEDNESDAY
THURSDAY
FRIDAY
SATURDAY
NOTES

HERBAL RECIPE PLANNER

DATE :

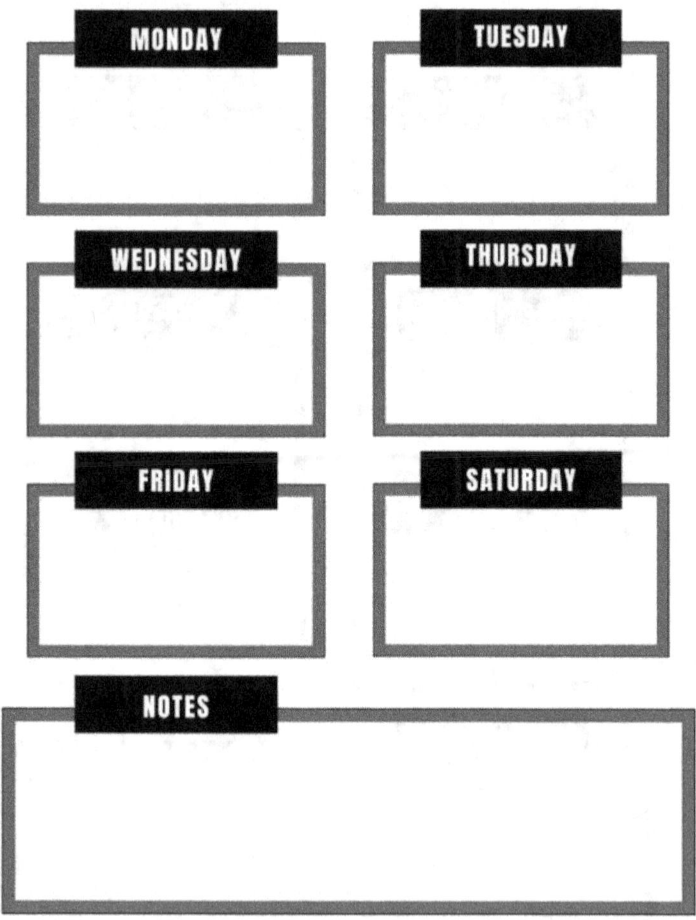

HERBAL RECIPE PLANNER

DATE :

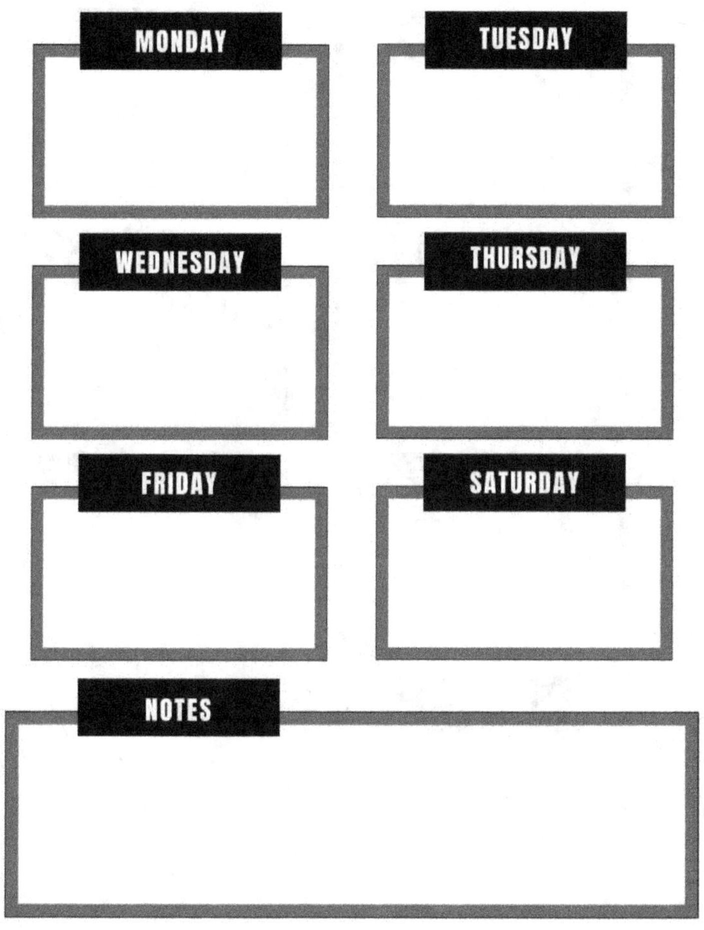

HERBAL RECIPE PLANNER

DATE :

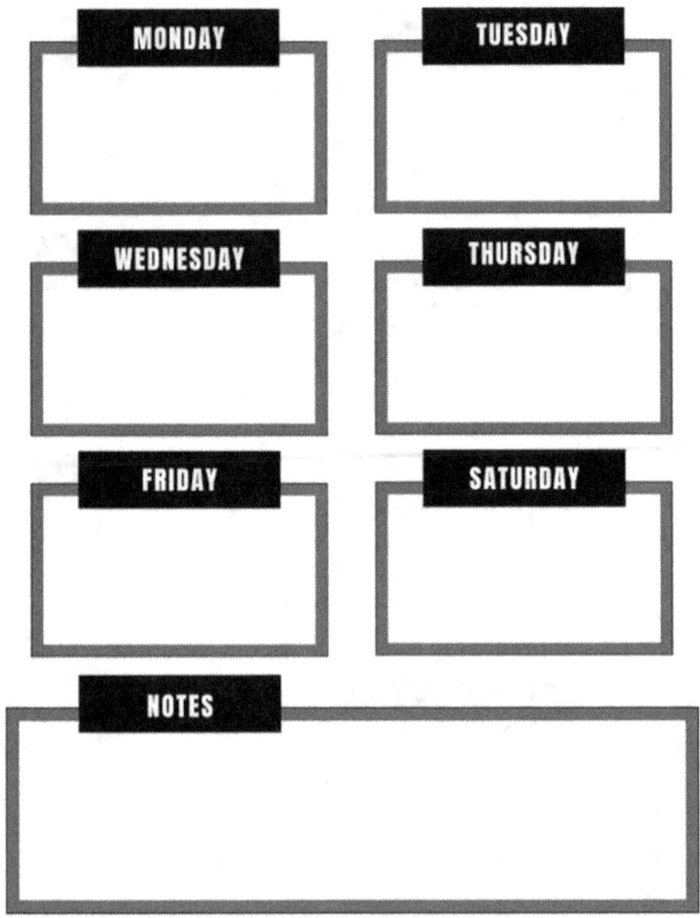

HERBAL RECIPE PLANNER

DATE :

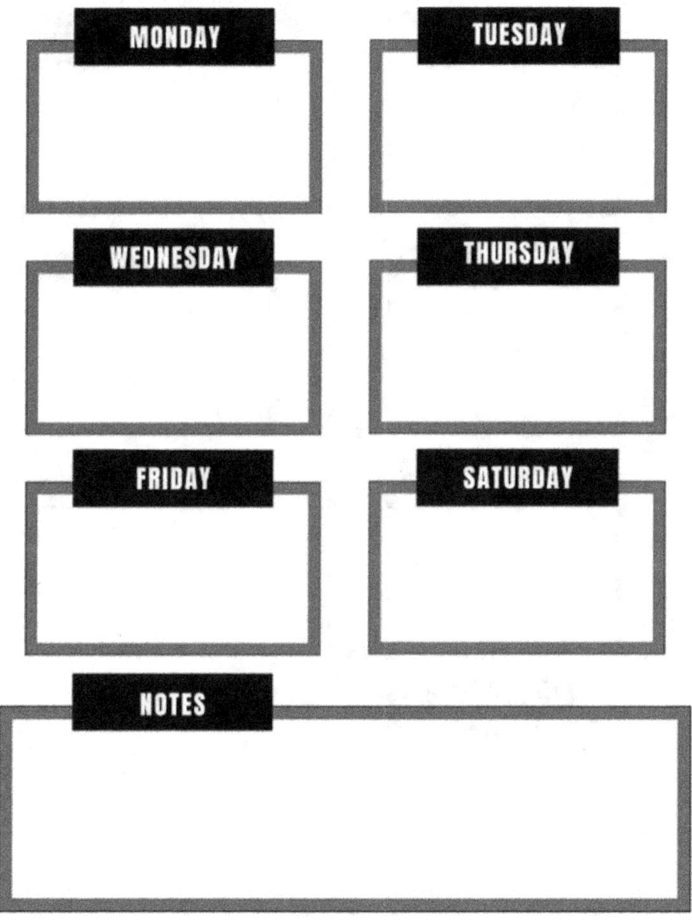

HERBAL RECIPE PLANNER

DATE :

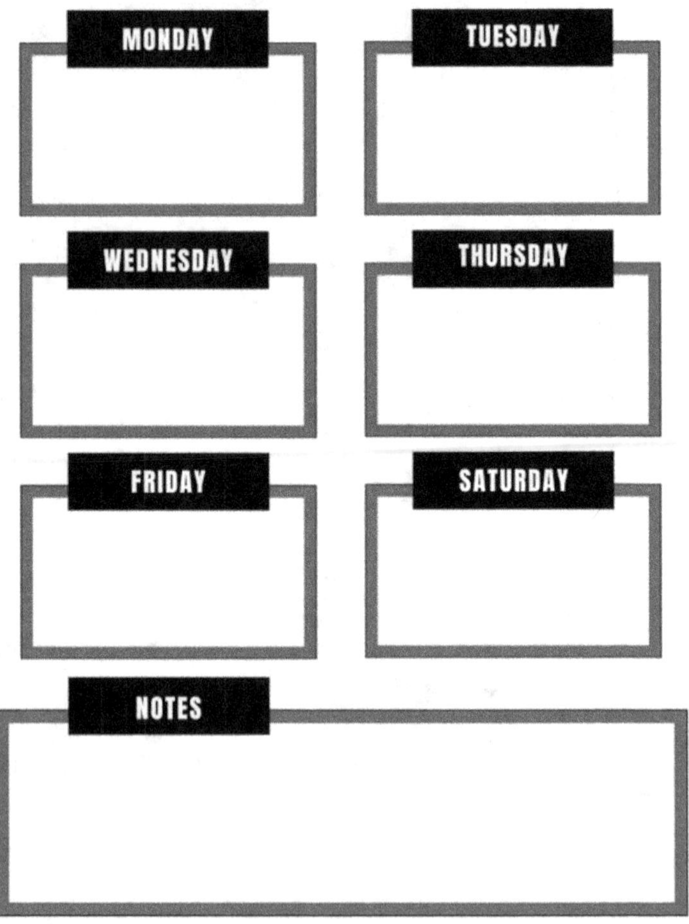

HERBAL RECIPE PLANNER

DATE :

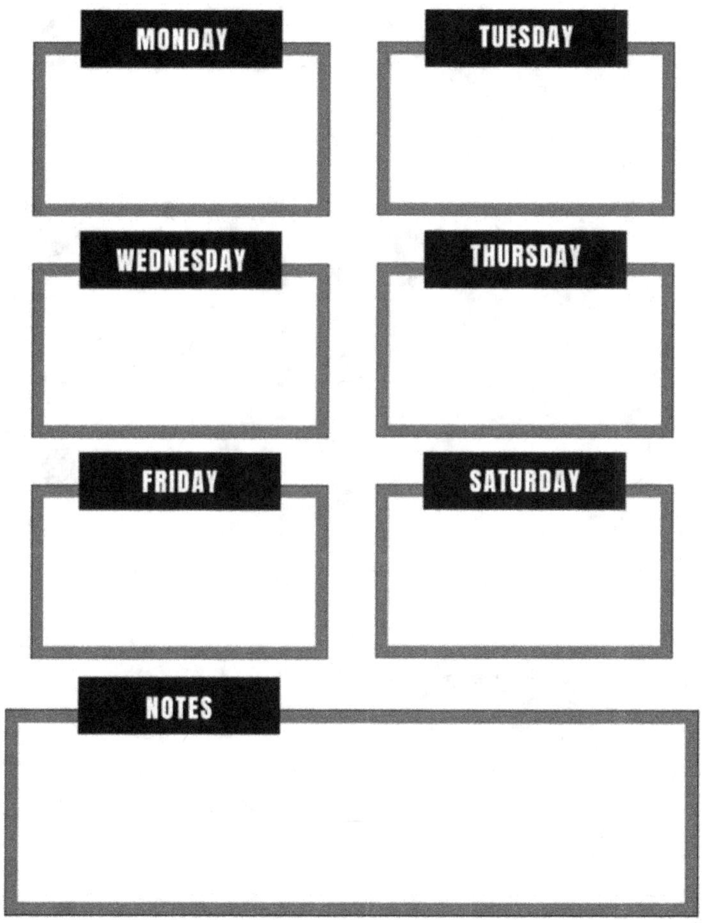

HERBAL RECIPE PLANNER

DATE :

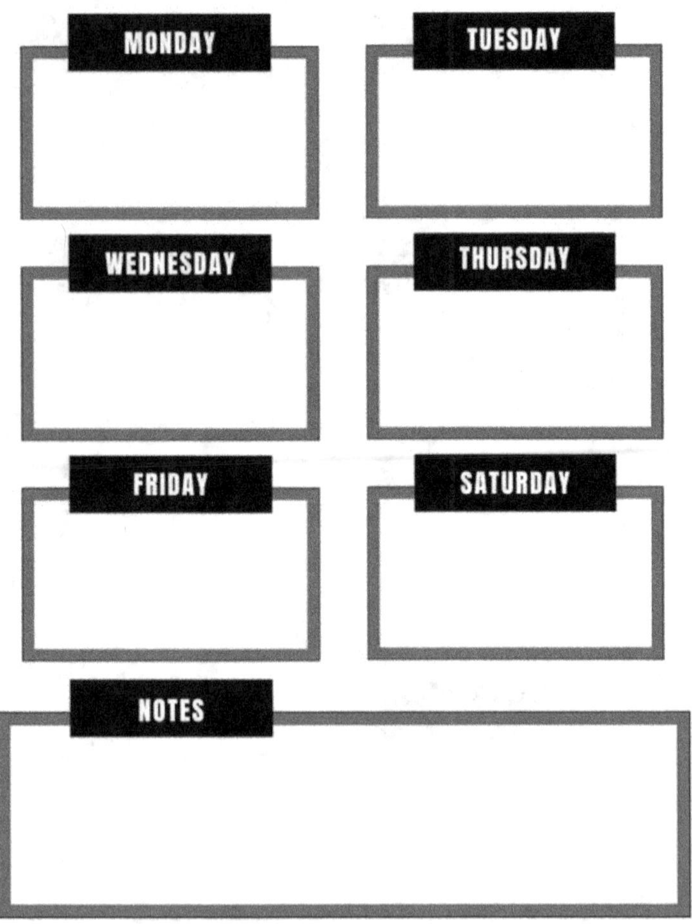